Contents

Weight Mastery

How To Condition Your Body To SHRED Fat With A Simple Guide

Introduction:
Why am I not losing weight?

It's a common story – you work out, eat right, your weight fluctuates by a couple of pounds and bounces right back, you give up. Frustrating isn't it? There's a huge reason why you're not getting anywhere. Most people don't know much at all about the actual science of weight-loss, and because of this you're almost guaranteed to sabotage yourself.

When you first start to work out or change your diet your body needs time to adjust. At first all you're going to lose is water weight, but similarly, if you're not drinking enough your body is going to compensate by holding water. Then your newly-exercised muscles are also going to hold water as they repair themselves.

Despite what you may think, your body is made up of a variety of different tissues. The most important ones for our purpose are muscle and fat. You may have heard that "muscle weighs more than fat", actually they both weigh the same but the muscle takes up less space and makes the body more efficient. When losing weight you want to retain as much muscle as possible.

Losing weight the wrong way means you're also losing muscle too and this can lower your metabolism.

The reason for this is that your muscle burns calories at a higher rate; the more muscle you have the more efficient your body is at burning calories. This doesn't mean you have to be a weightlifter to be thin, but it does mean that following in the same athletic steps can make your body leaner and more efficient.

Fat isn't just one single thing. Your body is made up of four distinct types of fat– white, brown, subcutaneous, and visceral. We need some body fat to survive, but the rest of it is what can damage our health. Brown fat can actually help you lose weight. People who are lean tend to have a higher brown fat to white fat ratio but it's also been shown that brown fat actually stimulates the body to lose white fat. Your body fat is only 2-3% brown fat. White fat, on the other hand, is where your body stores energy; it's usually what makes up what we consider "fat" to be – rolls, flab, etc. Subcutaneous fat sits directly under the skin and can be used to measure overall body fat. Subcutaneous fat doesn't cause as many problems as other types, unless it's located in the belly area. Visceral or abdominal fat is found around your inner organs and is a huge health problem. Unlike other types of fat you can't see this because it's inside you and even healthy people can still have a high level of visceral fat. It's thought that this type is responsible for insulin resistance and a risk of dementia. It's often the visceral fat that is the hardest to lose.

Similarly, you'll also find that body fat can exist in different areas. Some of the areas are more stubborn than others. Your thigh and buttock fat can actually be a good thing. It's been shown that women who have a higher (but still normal range) thigh and butt fat ratio are less likely to be affected by certain metabolic diseases. However, abdominal and belly fat are a health concern. Abdominal fat is linked to higher risks for a variety of diseases and it can drastically decrease your quality of life. When losing weight you'll find that you can't pick and choose, your body naturally loses fat from all over the body.

The great thing is that you can actually help your body a little. Your body is going to lose white fat first since it's in the highest quantity. Any weight loss will also help you with visceral fat but it won't make a huge difference overall. Exercise, on the other hand, has been shown to drastically improve the amount of visceral fat and belly fat lost. Combining both a proper diet and the right exercise regime will mean that your body loses more of the unsightly bulge and unhealthy fat.

So how can we burn the most white stuff while keeping the most muscle? Despite your efforts, you still might not have the right balance of working out and nutrition. Simply eating a calorie "amount" often isn't enough, and let's face it, it can also be woefully restrictive. You're starving to lose weight, and the moment you lose it you'll eat again and put it back on. It's a vicious circle.

Have you ever seen an athlete's diet? They can easily eat three or four times the calorie amount you can while still remaining sleek and lean. The reason for this is that their body is primarily muscle, and it's conditioned to power through fuel (food). Your body needs conditioning too if you want to be able to eat a full diet and lose weight at the same time. To get your body conditioned to lose fat rather than muscle you're going to have to have a good understanding of how it works.

Chapter 1:
Metabolism and diet

Your metabolism is key to losing weight, it is the process by which our bodies regulate the food we take in and how it's distributed. The body is a very efficient machine and it follows a simple equation:

Calories in + Calories out = Weight stored/lost

It honestly is that simple. The problem is counting calories is boring, and often it's hard to actually be precise enough to get it right. So, despite what some diets will tell you, it doesn't necessarily mean that what you eat matters as long as you're eating the right calorie number. The reason you *want* to care about what you're eating is because this isn't a very efficient way of thinking. If you're struggling to count calories, why would you want to make your life harder by adding junk food to it?

When our bodies metabolize food it is broken down into smaller nutrients and molecules to be used. Food is not just an energy source, it is used to rebuild, renew, and cleanse our body. Many athletes will tell you that "food is fuel"; it's actually so much more than that. Food is a comfort, it's memories, it's often just a way of not being bored. Similarly, food contains just as many nutrients and vitamins in it, or at least good food does.

The reason junk food is so bad for you is that it has very little nutritional value. Nutritional value is assigned based on how useful that food is to your body. Food can be broken down into three macronutrients – Protein, Carbohydrate and Fat. For 30 years the diet industry told us that eating fat will make us fat.

The problem was the food industry found that fat-free foods were tasteless so they loaded them up with sugar instead. Despite eating a fat-free diet, we got fatter.

Your body does different things with each macronutrient and most diet plans are based around one or more of these macronutrients. Low-cab, high-carb, protein only and high-fat. There are many different ones out there.

When we digest food our bodies break it down into macronutrients first. Carbohydrates are the most misunderstood macronutrient as you'll hear opposing arguments saying that they are both good and bad. Carbohydrates come in two forms – simple and complex. Simple carbohydrates are broken down quickly and cause your blood sugar to spike rapidly. They're meant as a quick form of energy. Complex carbohydrates break down slower and cause a more gradual rise. Your body uses carbs for a quick burst of energy, but if we don't use all the energy our body stores the remainder for later as body fat. If we don't have enough readily available energy our bodies turn to protein for sustenance.

High-protein diets have also been somewhat controversial; the reason for this is that too high a protein intake can be toxic to the body. The body processes proteins in the same way as carbohydrates, but the energy is much longer lasting and the excess protein is used within the body rather than converted into fat (usually). Protein is used in hair, skin, nail, and muscles. In fact, our bodies need protein after a workout to rebuild the tears in the muscle fibers caused by exercise. Protein is often lower in calories than other macronutrients but it can also be less nutrient dense. Eating excess protein will still make you fat, it just happens slower. So, eating fat has to be better right?

The fallacy about fat making you fat has made many cringe away from it. Fat is challenging because, like carbohydrates, it is higher in calories than protein. It's a lot easier to put on weight eating a high fat diet than it is to lose it. The problem is that a high-fat diet is extremely efficient and is an ideal way of losing weight. Fats can be good or bad because they come in so many forms. You've certainly heard about bad trans-fats and saturated fats, perhaps you've even heard of mono and poly-unsaturated fats. Good fats are used by the body for brain processes, hair, heart health and more while the bad fats either have to be excreted or stored until the body can use them for energy.

Athletes eat a very specific ratio of these macronutrients to have a lean, low fat, silhouette. The right fuel is imperative for their training, and without it they wouldn't be in the great shape that they are. Athlete's bodies are conditioned to burn fat for fuel rather than storing it because they burn it off so fast. You're going to need to do the same if you want to shred as much weight as possible.

Chapter 2:
Fix Your Diet for Fat-loss

There are a variety of dos and don'ts that come with eating like an athlete. Athlete's bodies are efficient; they burn calories at an astonishing rate because they have to. To eat like an athlete, you need a healthy diet that has sufficient nutrients and fuel. What you eat and drink matters. You'll need to eat a diet that gives your body the fuel and nutrients it needs without excess.

The first DO is to eat breakfast. Olympians always eat breakfast. When your body processes calories it produces the hormone insulin; if you don't eat those calories first thing your body won't start producing that hormone until later in the day. What this will do is it will actually lower your ability to process calories so you'll end up storing more fat. A good protein like egg whites, grass-fed dairy or high-protein grains is a good start. Avoid sugar, processed foods, and high-fat as these will cause a rapid insulin spike without giving you the lasting effects. Another important factor here is that you want to eat a large breakfast because it will stop you from binging on snack foods later, and it will also make you less hungry at the end of the day. A good estimate is 500-700 calories for breakfast.

Your diet also needs to have the right macro balance. Studies have shown that to improve fat-loss you'll need to limit the amount of carbohydrates you eat, and try to eliminate as many processed carbohydrates as much as possible. If you're going to rely on a low calorie diet to lose fat you're also going to end up losing muscle too, so instead of trying to starve yourself into losing weight, which we'll show later is going to actually give you the reverse, you'll need to eat adequate calories while still providing your body with proper nutrition. Long workouts require carbohydrates because your body needs the energy;

the problem is that these aren't going to help you burn off the body fat. On the other hand, if you're doing a shorter and more intense workout a high protein diet can provide just what is needed for maximum fat-loss.

The second is hydration; an estimated 75% of Americans suffer from chronic dehydration. This means that you're actively putting your body into a state where it's not functioning properly because you don't consume enough water. Don't confuse juice and soda with water. Water, coffee, and tea without anything added to them are the best thing for hydration. They're 0 calories, no added, sugar, and the right brands are also chemical and toxin free. Despite knowing we need our "8 glasses", few of us actually get them. Drinking water throughout the day is essential because through water our body flushes out toxins, waste products, and FAT.

If you want your body to let go of the excess fat it has to have a method of getting rid of it. Poop is 80% water; without having enough water our bodies cannot let go of the waste products our metabolism produces. 8 glasses of water are often not enough for most people, especially those overweight. You might find you actually need double that at first!

On top of all this, you still need to eat well. If you're not getting the right nutrient density, then your body is at risk for a variety of malnutrition diseases. Many high-protein diets insist you take a multivitamin for this exact reason – you're not getting adequate nutrients from your food. The priority here is to stop snacking. We're bombarded with adverts and social suggestions to snack, 50-60 years ago there was no such thing. Snacking is an ideal way to boost your calories, or put you over your calorie amount. Many snacks are sugary, sodium filled, or just plain nutrient duds.

Eat 3-4 good sized meals a day, drink adequate water, and you'll find that you don't need to snack. Many times our snacking is a mistaken need for water. Have a glass of water instead and then decide if you're still hungry. With your meals, you'll need to get the right nutrients. Focus on eating fat. This doesn't mean eating a slab of butter for dinner but foods that are rich in good fats are usually also high in protein. Grass-fed meat, eggs, fish, cheese, nuts, seeds, olive oil, avocado and even coconut are all rich in good fats.

Most nutritionists recommend an intake that is 50% carbohydrate, 20-30% fat and 20-30% protein. The reason for this is that 50% is the magic carbohydrate number. If you eat more than this your body will likely not be getting enough protein or your body is going to store it instead of burning through it. If you eat less than 50% carbohydrate a lot of the time your body will convert proteins into carbohydrates to balance the process back out. Egg whites are a perfect example of this as your body will take the protein from them and process them as a carbohydrate if your carbohydrate count is too low. Getting a food tracker or keeping a diet diary is an ideal way of learning how to do this so that it eventually becomes instinctual.

Finally, you'll also need to follow the right routine to promote ultimate fat loss. If you've tried weight-loss before you'll know how hard it is not to end up stuck in a rut with the same schedule week after week. You're going to find that this routine is your enemy when it comes to losing the maximum amount of fat. If you're determined to do the same routine exercise over and over again while on a low-calorie diet your body is also going to lose muscle. This will inhibit its ability to burn calories and ultimately will also stall your weight loss. What you want to do is to make sure that you're only losing fat instead of both muscle and fat together.

Chapter 3:
Lose Fat instead of Muscle

Now that you know what to eat it's time to learn how to make sure that your body is at its most efficient to put that to good use. Having a great diet won't make you lean, it might make you thinner overall but it's not going to shred fat fast. First you're going to want to calculate how much you should weigh. This can be quite a subjective matter; height, genetics, muscle composition are all factors that can influence these numbers. Have you ever heard people that say they are "big boned"? Well their skeleton is the same size but their lean muscle/fat ratio might be higher. What you're looking for is the optimum level of fat/muscle. This will vary mostly by your athleticism and gender as you can see from this table:

	Athlete	Healthy	Overweight
Men 20-29	3-10%	15-18%	20%+
Men 30-39	5-12%	14-22%	23%+
Men 40-49	6-15%	15-24%	26%+
Men 50+	8-17%	19-28%	30%+
Women 20-29	10-16%	17-27%	29%+
Women 30-39	11-17%	20-29%	30%+

Women 40-49	13-20%	24-33%	34%+
Women 50+	14-22%	26-36%	37%+

You'll need these three equations to figure out your ideal weight:

Body fat mass = current weight x current body fat percentage

Lean body mass = current weight – fat mass

Goal weight = current lean body mass ÷ goal lean body mass

You'll likely only reach the lowest end of the spectrum if you're strict, exercise hard and lose weight easily. Most athletes don't consider themselves to be at their lowest and are constantly trying to shed more body fat. With the wrong nutrition you're going to lose lean body mass, so what you want to be doing is building muscle at the same time as losing fat. It's a very delicate balance. Even a few pounds more of lean muscle can mean a huge difference in calorie burn.

The right workout is almost as important as your diet when it comes to losing fat instead of muscle. Look at different athletes – runners are lean, thin, svelte and they burn a ton of calories; while weightlifters are bulky, thick, muscular and still burn a ton of calories. Both bodies are efficient, but they have entirely different shapes. You'll need to work with a workout combination that gives you the result you want. More cardio/more weights, either way it's important to do both or you'll find you're losing muscle mass as well and your weight-loss will slow or even plateau off. If you've ever tried losing weight you're well aware of the dreaded plateau.

The plateau is that wall many people hit after losing a portion of weight where you just can't seem to get past it and keep going. You're stuck. Maybe you're there already which is why you've bought this book. To avoid a plateau or to get off it you have to shake things up. Scientists used to say that fat loss was all about long, slow, starved, cardio exercises. In fact, it can have the opposite effect, you'll end up burning muscle as well as fat. Now we know that it isn't about what burns the most fat during each training session but how to optimize your body to burn the most fat for each 24-hour period. HIIT, which means short, high-intensity, workouts have been touted as the ideal solution to this problem.

HIIT is a short, but intense, exercise period that creates an oxygen debt in the muscles. The muscles continue to burn oxygen long after you've finished exercising which means your metabolic boost will last long after you're done training. The problem here is you can still plateau on HIIT. You'll need to switch it up as needed with strength training and strength conditioning to stop your body getting stuck in a rut. You'll also need to allow for stretching, and give your muscles time to rest and rebuild.

But what if your body is efficient already? Sometimes we're doing great at being healthy but our fat just wants to be stubborn. There's often a reason for this. Stress releases a hormone called cortisol which causes the body to hang on to, and even store more fat! If you're stressed, you'll sometimes find it's impossible to lose fat no matter how hard you try. Stubborn fat is often a side effect of negative stress in your life.

Stubborn fat can also be physiologically different than regular fat. Most cells have connectors on them, a bit like Lego or Meccano, so that they can join with other cells. Fat cells are no different. Once these cells bond with another using receptors the bond can be very difficult to break. When it comes to weight-loss you only need to concern yourself with alpha-2 and beta-2 receptors. The ratio of the 2 receptors is what determines how hard a fat cell is to release from its bonded state. The more alpha-2 receptors a cell has, the more difficult it is to break off. Women tend to have more alpha-2 receptors in their fat than men, but physiologically they actually are allowed more fat in their normal range than men in the "stubborn" areas. So how can we get rid of something that's built in?

The key is to mess with that bond; since the beta-2 receptors aren't an issue you'll want them to keep functioning while getting the alpha-2 receptors to let go. Your secret weapon is a hormone called catecholamine. Epinephrine and norepinephrine are produced in response to stress, technically the stress of exercise also produces these but it's mostly in response to anxiety. HIIT conveniently produces a greater amount of catecholamine. Keeping your insulin level low is a good way of keeping the beta-2 receptors active while leaving the alpha-2 ones "asleep" if you will. Even a small insulin increase can energize those alpha-2 receptors again which is why a high-protein diet is so important. It fuels your body without spiking your insulin levels suddenly. A protein-rich, low-glycemic diet, combined with HIIT exercise is the ideal way to power through even the most stubborn fat cells.

The biggest tip for fat-loss with exercise is NOT to follow a program. Those easy to get DVD systems, the work-out plans, the meal plans. STOP. Real fat-loss training will have you forgetting what day of the week is leg day, building calluses from lifting an adequate weight, and have your body in a state where it constantly loses fat because it isn't getting used to the same exercises over and over again. When burning fat, you should rotate your exercise conditioning between short and intense workouts and longer conditioning work to get your body burning fat instead of muscle.

Combining the right workout with proper nutrition is the only way you'll get your body to its most efficient fat burning state.

Chapter 4:
BUSTED: Myths of Metabolism

BUSTED: Weight Training makes you Thick

Getting stronger is an important part of becoming lean, if you fail to do strength training your body will also lose lean muscle mass and you'll find your weight loss slowing down. Ultimately, if you have more lean muscle mass you'll also be able to burn more calories (and therefore take more calories in). The better you are with strength training the better level you will be at other training and this will make your body more effective at getting rid of the excess body fat. You'll help your metabolism by keeping your body's ability to burn calories higher with weight training.

BUSTED: Extremes will reach your goal faster

Working your body hard is great, but it can actually be negative too. You need to work your body smart instead. Over-training is what happens when you work out too much, you risk injury, damage, and can stall your weight-loss by overtiring your muscles without adequate rest. The same applies to extreme calorie restriction. If you eat too little for the training level you're at your body will enter starvation mode. This is where your body tries to store every calorie you take in just to survive. Your metabolism slows and any excess calories are quickly packed on as fat to be used when the starvation period happens again. This is what happens with extreme yo-yo diets.

BUSTED: You have to follow a specific diet to lose fat

Calories in – Calories out. The process is simple. You will lose weight just following this theory, but you won't be at your most efficient to lose fat, and you'll probably lose at a slower rate than you could. To lose fat effectively, you need to know your macronutrients and your ratios. As long as you're within those numbers your body, an efficient machine, can do the rest. Remember to take nutrient density into account to make sure you're not at risk of malnutrition. Your metabolism runs very efficiently, but you can definitely help it out by eating well.

BUSTED: Skipping breakfast and fasting make it easier

When you're not eating your metabolism slows down. By fasting and skipping breakfast your metabolism doesn't recover, it stays down for the rest of the day. Eating a healthy breakfast will boost your metabolism and get your day started right so that your body burns calories at a higher rate and shreds your body fat. Start your body with a good amount of protein which will help you burn calories without letting you get hungry fast.

BUSTED: Caffeine amps up your metabolism

No. The sugar in most caffeine filled drinks will amp up your body fat though. Caffeine does provide a slight boost to your metabolism, but most caffeinated drinks are stuffed with toxins, sugars, and junk. The typical energy drink has a quarter of your day's sugar allowance or more in it. Plain coffee and tea are the only exceptions. If you're struggling to drink plain water consider flavoring it with slices of lemon, a known metabolism booster, or choose unsweetened, freshly-made tea.

BUSTED: 1lb of muscle burns 100 calories a day

It's no secret that muscle is more efficient at burning fat/calories, but simply breaking it into an equation like that doesn't work. Muscle does burn calories at a higher rate than fat just to exist but the rate also fluctuates based on resistance exercise, cardio, rest etc. Your brain tissue in comparison actually does burn at that rate. So if you work on building the gray matter in your brain you'll actually burn 109 calories a day for a pound of brain matter. As long as you're exercising you're still burning calories and it's also shown to improve brain function!

BUSTED: Working out on an empty stomach burns more calories

Before a workout you shouldn't be over-full but your stomach should also not be empty. It's a good idea to consume a protein rich snack because it will give your body fuel without giving it too much carbohydrate. Don't take a big glass of water before either but remember to hydrate during exercise.

BUSTED: All fat is bad

Your body needs a minimum amount of fat just to survive. Your brain, for example, is fatty tissue. Sometimes when you're already in the healthy and lean zone you'll find an area that's stubborn. This area might just be something you'll need to live with. Even top athletes have a percentage of body fat, it's just lower than the average person. Remember the alpha and beta receptors? Are you more stressed than you wish to accept? Think about what's going on in your life and whether your body might be hanging on to that last stubborn bit for a reason beyond diet and exercise.

Chapter 5:
Getting Prepped

Athlete's bodies are well-conditioned machines; if you're reading this there's a good chance that your body is far from that. The problem for most people is getting started, taking the first step is often the hardest but saying you're going to go to the gym burns 0 calories while actually going is what you need to be doing. It's all very well that you've got the information but you'll actually need to follow it through. We've talked about setting a reasonable weight-loss goal, but once you've set the goals you'll have to actually do them. If you've never done any form of exercise before check-in with your doctor first to make sure there ares no health reasons you're not ready for exercise. They may also give you suggestions on methods or a prescription to help you get started.

Motivating your brain is just as important as conditioning your body. Making your goals public and plotting your progress once you get started are ideal ways of staying on track. You'll feel more inclined to actually do things if other people know about it. You can even reward yourself when you reach mini-goals like 20% body fat, 15% body fat etc. Try not to reward yourself with food since it's counterproductive. Consider new gym shoes, or a relaxing massage.

When you're getting ready to work out it's important to stretch your muscles beforehand. Warming your muscles up is key because you might get cramp otherwise. Not only this but exciting the muscles and nervous system means that your workout will be more productive. Foam rollers, light yoga, stretches, a short walk, anything that makes your body feel warm without too much effort is an ideal way to warm-up your body for maximum fat loss during your workout. If you're just getting started your warm-up might be as far as you can manage for the first few days; remember pushing yourself to an extreme is simply setting your body up for damage. Start slow, your body didn't gain the weight overnight so it's not going to lose it overnight either.

Here are some suggestions on meals to eat before working out that are designed for ultimate fat loss:

Cheesy Skillet Eggs

Eggs are an ideal food for protein, and the added dairy can also bump up the protein amount. Cook them in an iron skillet for added iron while you're at it. Eggs are also high in vitamin D which can help boost your breathing and choline, a nutrient known for its anti-anxiety properties. Avoid adding salt as it negatively affects blood pressure.

Ingredients:

- 3 eggs

- ¼ cups shredded cheese

- 1 green onion, thinly sliced

- 1tbs coconut Oil

- Pepper to taste

Directions: Whisk eggs and cheese together and set aside. In the skillet melt the coconut oil. Add the green onion and sauté for 1 minute. Add the egg mixture and fold over until eggs are cooked through. Serve immediately on a low-carb wrap or on their own.

Yoghurt with Fruitola

Greek yoghurt is packed with protein (check the sugar content though). Adding a small amount of seeds or granola is an ideal way to boost this while adding healthy fats and fiber. A small serving of berries can help sweeten it and also add fiber. Choose fresh fruit as most dried fruit is soaked in sugar before drying.

Ingredients:

- 1 cup Greek yoghurt

- ¼ cup granola (or substitute for equal measure of 1 tbsp. chia seed, 1 tbsp. unsweetened shredded coconut, and 1 tbsp. slivered almonds)

- ¼ cup sliced strawberries

Directions: In a bowl (or in the pot if your yoghurt is pre-measured) layer the granola and top with berries. Serve immediately.

Protein Smoothie

Smoothies and juicing have gotten a lot of PR recently; they are an ideal way to eat a small meal on the go but can still pack a big nutritional punch. A smoothie has the added benefit of the fiber from any fruits and vegetables which makes it preferable to juicing. Choosing Kefir over milk adds a protein punch.

Ingredients:

- ½ cup plain kefir

- ½ cup frozen strawberries

- 2tbsp. peanut butter

- 1 frozen banana

- 2tbsp. walnuts

- Ice cubes to adjust consistency

Directions: Place all the ingredients into a blender and pulse until smooth.

HIGH PROTEIN PRE-WORKOUT SNACKS:

If you're working out between meals choosing a high-protein snack can be just as effective. Remember to measure in accordingly with your calories so try not to think of this as a whole meal.

Protein Popsicle

A great treat in the summer, this can be a perfect way to get your workout going with only one hand to spare.

Ingredients:

- 1 cup unsweetened chocolate almond milk (or kefir)

- 1 scoop chocolate protein powder

- 2tbsp. unsweetened cocoa powder

- 2 tbsp. peanut butter

Directions: Blend ingredients together and pour into popsicle molds. Leave about a ½ inch at the top since they will expand. Freeze at least 6 hours before eating.

Yoghurt Berries

These can also be an ideal snack food since they're very low in calories and quite filling. If you find them too tart add a few drops of stevia or monk fruit extract to the yoghurt first to sweeten it. For an added protein boost have a spoonful of nut butter with them.

Ingredients:

- ½ cup Greek yoghurt

- 1/3 cup blueberries

Directions: Line a cookie sheet with baking paper and place close by. In a bowl combine the yoghurt and sweetener, if needed. Using a toothpick carefully impale a blueberry and dip it into the yoghurt, using another slide the blueberry off onto the pan. Make sure you do this gently so it doesn't roll. Repeat for all blueberries. Put the pan into the freezer for 2 hours, retrieve, and tip all the blueberries into an airtight bag. Store on the door/top of the freezer as this tends to be the warmest part. Eat straight from the freezer!

SUPPLEMENTS:

Many people will tell you there is no magic pill for fat-loss. In fact, the diet industry makes billions each year selling a variety of magic pills "guaranteed" to help you achieve your weight-loss goals. Most of them don't work. It is still your metabolism and your body's own processes that will ultimately make you lose weight through the calorie equation. However, that isn't to say that you can't give it a little bit of help to make sure it's burning nothing but fat. Stimulants are commonly thought of as the best fat burners, but they're also risky as they can cause you to have heart problems, palpitations and can also upset your digestive system. Try and look for natural supplements or insist on ones that are stimulant free. Always consult your doctor before adding any supplements to avoid clashes with medication; they may even be able to suggest some.

Garcinia Cambogia

Made from the Malabar Tamarind fruit, the fruit contains an acid (hydroxycitric acid) that has been popular as a supplement for almost 20 years. Since 2012 studies have rapidly accumulated supporting it as one of the best fat-loss supplements available, and it's legal. HCA is an ideal tool in your arsenal to boost your fat loss. The reason for this is that it blocks an enzyme which turns sugar into fat; because of this carbohydrate can then be used as fuel since the body is unable to store as fat. It's also been shown to have limited appetite suppressing qualities. Look for a supplement that has at least 50% HCA as well as potassium or magnesium. It's important that you take it 30-60 minutes before eating to allow the enzyme to kick in or it won't work.

Green Coffee Bean

Before coffee beans are roasted they are in fact green. Dr. Oz made them much more popular recently but they've been around for a while. Coffee beans contain a variety of antioxidants including chlorogenic acids. These lower blood pressure and promote weight loss. A good supplement is at least 45% Chlorogenic acid but, be aware that many cheap products use fillers and chemicals to thin the product and make more money. Try not to overdo these supplements as they are somewhat of a stimulant (much like a cup of coffee). The reason coffee doesn't have the same effect is that the roasting process greatly reduces the chlorogenic acid content.

Raspberry Ketones

Ketones are something your body naturally produces; you may have heard of the ketogenic diet. Another supplement made famous by Dr. Oz, raspberry ketones are often called a "miracle fat burner". The reason for this is that ketones have been linked to being able to break through the weight-loss plateau. 100-200mg of ketone supplement twice a day can help avoid the block. Ketones work by regulating norepinephrine in the body, which we've already seen can cause you to gain or hold fat because of stress. It also causes a spike in body temperature which helps with fat-loss. Unlike other supplements though raspberry ketones come with more health warnings, they are linked to asthma, heart and blood sugar issues.

Some Suggested Supplements:

Evlution Nutrition's Leanmode

Rated as one of the top exercise supplements Leanmode is a stimulant free supplement that offers 5 boosts to help you lose more fat. The supplement contains many of the most popular additives as well as adding in amino acids that support the utilization of fat cells as fuel during workouts.

Hydroxycut Hardcore

Hydroxycut is one of the most well-known brands out there, they've been around a long time and have a huge selection of products to choose from. The hardcore formula is a sustained release product that has been designed to promote thermogenesis. Thermogenesis is a raising of body temperature; it occurs naturally during exercise but you can also use a supplement to boost it. It is NOT stimulant-free but has been shown to produce good results.

RSP QuadraLean

Another stimulant-free choice this has only 4 of the main fat-loss boosts but relies on amino acids and thermogenesis in the brown fat to work properly. It uses the most popular supplement ingredients and works efficiently like most other good quality supplements.

Once your body is primed and ready to go you can start looking at exercises to get maximum fat-loss. Remember it's not a race so starting on a slower rate and building up is what will get your body burning calories like an athlete rather than burning them off and packing them back on.

Chapter 6:
Building up to HIIT Work-outs

Now that your body is all fueled up you'll need the right workout regimen to burn maximum fat. As mentioned, you'll need to keep your body confused so that it doesn't plateau. Each of these workouts can be switched around, combined or skipped for rest days so your body is constantly in a state of flux. Remember to include rest days in any regimen so you don't risk over training.

HIIT should be done in moderation – between rest days and moderate days, to avoid a massive increase in muscle mass. HIIT can cause you to bulk up if it's used too often so use it only between your other workouts so that this doesn't happen. If you suddenly find yourself gaining after adding in HIIT to your schedule cut back and maybe do 1 or 2 sessions less a week. Ideally you only need 1-2 a week anyway but if you want maximum fat-loss you need to build up to doing at least 20-30 minutes. If you can't do these workouts right off start without doing the repeats and build up. As you can see they're all easily broken down so try and build up to doing the whole thing. Your early conditioning might seem slow and painful but remember, you're preparing your body to lose the fat fast and keep it off.

HIIT Exercises

Time 15 minutes approx.

Workout-1:

10 burpees + 10 mountain climbers + 10 jumping jacks

15 burpees + 15 mountain climbers + 15 jumping jacks

20 burpees + 20 mountain climbers + 20 jumping jacks

3 minutes jump rope

1 minute rest (rehydrate)

45 seconds lunges

15 second break

45 seconds pushups

15 second break

45 seconds lunge jumps

 15 second break

45 seconds inchworms

3 minutes jump rope

FINISH

Workout-2:

45 second kettlebell squats

15 second break

45 second pull-ups

15 second break

45 second box jumps

15 second break

45 second pushups

3 minutes jump rope

1 minute rest

Repeat

45 seconds side lunges

15 second break

45 seconds dips

15 second break

45 second speed skaters

15 second break

45 second pushups

Repeat x2

FINISH

Workout-3:

20 seconds jump rope

10 second break

20 second push up

10 second break

20 second bodyweight rows

10 second break

20 second burpee

10 second break

20 second plank

10 second break

20 second lunges

10 second break

1 minute jump rope

Rest 1 minute

Repeat x 2

FINISH

Conclusion:
Keeping the Fat away

So you've actually done it! Your high-protein/HIIT combo has actually shifted even the stubborn fat you tried to lose. Congratulations, this is the hardest part – keeping it off. Many people who diet swiftly find themselves back on the treadmill because they've gained weight *again*. The reason for this is that you need to make this a lifestyle change and not just a temporary weight-loss program.

Look at your lifestyle – do you have a sedentary job, are you guilty of sitting on the couch watching television too much, have you stopped working out now you've reached your goal? Making a lifestyle change is key to keeping the fat at bay. You'll need to look at maintenance calories rather than weight-loss levels and continue to be aware of portion size. If your day is sedentary adjust your calories accordingly. A healthy lifestyle will stop you gaining it back on, you can't simply return to the old one and hope it won't come back because it doesn't work like that.

Remember the calories in-calories out equation? It will still apply when you've reached your goals. You can probably introduce more carbohydrates into your diet now since your maintenance calories will be a little higher than your loss calories (but not too high or you'll gain).

Choose appropriate supplements, eat the right amount, and exercise accordingly and not only will you lose the weight fast but you'll also have the tools to keep it off for life!

Hopefully you've learned a little about how your body works and how to get it in the perfect condition to burn fat in the fastest way possible while still conditioning it to keep the fat away long-term.

There are many fictional things about weight-loss out there, don't listen to them! Know your body and how it works and you'll have the magic key to being a leaner, thinner, and more confident you!

Kindly leave a review on what you enjoyed most about this book. That would really help me out greatly in my future publications.

www.ingramcontent.com/pod-product-compliance
Lightning Source LLC
Chambersburg PA
CBHW071319280526
45788CB00004B/1953